# Transformation journey for Tony Hudgell

A Remarkable Tale of Courage, Resilience, and Hope as a Double-Amputee Boy Faces Life-Changing Surgery

## Sam Gastel

# Copyright

# Table of Content

# Tony Hudgell's Incredible Adventure

There are hardly many tales of human tenacity as remarkable as Tony Hudgell's. Tony was born into a world where violence and suffering were commonplace, yet his path serves as evidence of the human spirit's unwavering ability to overcome hardship.

Tony, who is just nine years old, has already seen more adversity than most people would in their lifetime, yet his steadfast will and contagious positivity are a source of inspiration for everyone who hears his story.

Tony's tale starts with a terrible chapter filled with unspeakable violence and treachery. He lost both of his legs as a newborn as a consequence of horrifying maltreatment he endured from his birth parents.

The physical wounds from this horrible deed served as a continual reminder of the anguish and suffering he had to go through in his early years. However, Tony's spirit never wavered, a glimmer of hopefulness amid the shadows, even at the darkest moments.

Tony's adoptive family served as his beacon of hope throughout this difficult period. They gave Tony a second shot at life and the opportunity to change his tale, welcoming him as their own with unconditional love and support. Tony found comfort and strength under the tender care of Paula Hudgell, his adoptive mother, and set out on a path of recovery and self-discovery.

Even though Tony's illness limited his movement, he refused to let it define him. Refusing to allow his surroundings determine his destiny, he repeatedly defeated the odds with unwavering tenacity and resolve.

His contagious grin and unbreakable attitude made him amiable to everyone in his path and encouraged numerous others to keep going in the face of hardship.

However, Tony's adventure was far from ended. Driven by a fierce ambition to restore his self-reliance, he aimed for a significant objective: being able to walk without the need of crutches.

He put himself through physically taxing treatment sessions for years, pushing himself to achieve his goal. And at last, his persistence was rewarded. Tony started a life-altering surgical odyssey that would redefine what it means to defy the odds, all with the help of his committed medical team.

With wonder and adoration, the entire globe watches Tony at Sheffield Children's Hospital getting ready for his next surgery.

His tale is a potent reminder of the human spirit's resiliency and a ray of hope in a world all too frequently clouded by gloom. Tony approaches the path ahead with unflinching optimism and resolve, despite the fact that it may be filled with obstacles.

Tony Hudgell is a brilliant example of bravery, resiliency, and optimism in the face of hardship. His incredible journey is proof of the human spirit's ability to prevail even in the most trying situations.

We can only be in awe of the amazing young man he has grown into and the limitless possibilities that lies ahead as he starts this new chapter in his life.

# The Tragic Beginnings: Triumphing Against Misery

A small boy's life was irrevocably changed by a catastrophe that occurred in the calm areas of West Malling, Kent. Tony Hudgell came into the world full of purity and unbounded promise, but the darkness of human brutality quickly cast a shadow over his path.

Tony's biological parents subjected him to horrific maltreatment as a newborn, leaving him with scars that would follow him for years. Tony's early years were characterised by unspeakable misery and despair; the details of this horrific chapter are too agonising to describe.

More than just his physical health was taken from Tony by the assault; it also destroyed his feeling of security and faith in the outside world.

From people who ought to have shielded him, all he witnessed was brutality and treachery. But even at the lowest points of his suffering, Tony's spirit held firm, providing a ray of hope in the middle of despair.

The unexpected turn that Tony's narrative took occurred in the middle of this gloom. Through a strange turn of events, he was welcomed into a new family that was characterised by love and compassion rather than blood.

Tony was given a second shot at life and a chance to get past the scars of his past by his adopted parents, Paula and Mark Hudgell, who welcomed him into their home and hearts.

With the tender care of his new family, Tony started his protracted and difficult road to recovery. Physically, he had an arduous path ahead; his injuries were significant and his recuperation would take time and many obstacles.

However, the most challenging to heal were the emotional wounds. Tony suffered with feelings of dread, wrath, and betrayal for years as he attempted to reconcile with the trauma he had experienced in the past.

Nevertheless, Tony refused to let his circumstances define him, even in light of how great the challenges he faced. He set out on a path of rehabilitation and self-discovery with his family's steadfast support, aiming to regain his feeling of independence and self-worth.

After several hours of therapy and recovery, he gradually started to regain his strength and self-assurance, getting closer to normalcy every day.

The resiliency with which Tony overcame adversity, rather than the hardship itself, may have been the most impressive component of his journey.

Even after going through unspeakable anguish and suffering in his early years, Tony resisted giving up. Rather, he came out of the shadows with a renewed feeling of will and purpose, resolved to make the most out of his suffering.

Tony is full of hope and optimism despite his advanced age as he gets ready for his forthcoming operation. Despite the difficulties that lie ahead, he meets them head-on with bravery and resiliency because he is supported by a network of caring people and a loving family.

Tony Hudgell's tale is a potent reminder of the human potential for optimism and resilience in the face of unfathomable hardship.

Despite his unfortunate beginnings, he has had a triumphant path, which is a monument to the tenacious spirit that everyone of us possesses.

# A Glimmer of Hope: Gearing Up for Transformative Surgery

A little child is ready to go off on a voyage that would change his life forever in the middle of Sheffield's bustling city life. With a spirit as strong as steel, Tony Hudgell is about to embark on a significant new chapter in his incredible journey: an operation that will alter his life and change the definition of what it means to overcome adversity.

Tony's journey to this point has been filled with obstacles and hardships that would have tried the mettle of the most resilient people. He was born into a world filled with brutality and misery, and he suffered terrible torture at the hands of his biological parents, which left him without a limb. However, a small child whose unshakable bravery and unbounded optimism serve as an example to everyone who hears his tale rose from the ashes of tragedy.

Anticipation looms large as Tony gets ready for his impending operation at Sheffield Children's Hospital. This is the result of months of training that has brought him one step closer to his dream of being able to walk without the use of crutches.

Tony confronts the obstacles that lie ahead with the same determination and fortitude that have seen him through his darkest moments.

Paula Hudgell, Tony's adoptive mother, describes her journey up to this point as nothing less than an emotional rollercoaster. With a hint of trepidation mixed with enthusiasm, she continues, "We have been planning for this for almost the last year now." "We're a little bit nervous now because we know it's fast-approaching."

It's true that the thought of having such a major surgery may cause anyone's heart to rush with excitement. However, Tony's desire of being able to walk without crutches at last has gotten him through his worst moments. He says, "I want to run," with a resolve that defies his young age.

However, Tony and his family are well aware of the difficulties that may lie ahead as the operation day approaches. Tony will have to spend up to a year in a cage for his leg and hip throughout the taxing process of physical rehabilitation. But Tony is ready to take on any challenge because he has a steely resolve and his family's everlasting support.

Paula's path to this point has been fraught with several tense days and restless nights. "We thought we might have to travel to America for the surgery, which would have led to a huge amount of fundraising," she says. "But we have found one other person that can perform this operation, who works at Sheffield Children's Hospital."

Tony and his family are relieved to be able to have the procedure performed closer to home. Despite the fact that they would have to travel to Sheffield every week from London, they feel reassured and at ease knowing that the surgeon, Mr. James Fernandes, is a skilled professional who will handle the procedure.

Excitement builds as Tony's operation date draws nearer and nearer. With hope for Tony's future, friends and supporters from all around the world offer encouraging and supportive words.

Tony's narrative, which shines brilliantly even in the darkest of circumstances, is a striking reminder of the human spirit's perseverance in the face of hardship.

There's a calm resolve in the air the morning before Tony's operation as the sun rises over Sheffield Children's Hospital. Tony's life is about to change drastically, and Mr. Fernandes and his team are getting ready to start this adventure in the operating room.

And as Tony nods off to sleep, surrounded by his family's love and support, he knows that he will meet any problems head-on with the same bravery and tenacity that have brought him this far.

Tony Hudgell's path thus far has been one of tragedy over comeback, a monument to the strength of hope and will to get over even the most formidable challenges. And he does so knowing that he is not alone and that a community of love and support will be at his side every step of the way as he takes his first hesitant steps towards a future full of promise and opportunity.

# Overcoming Obstacles: The Path to Recuperation

Following a tragic event, Tony Hudgell's life took an unexpected turn that left him facing many challenges and uncertainties. He was born into a world filled with brutality and misery, and his biological parents subjected him to horrible violence that left him without a limb.

But a small child whose unflinching strength and tenacity would inspire countless others to endure in the face of hardship rose from the ashes of despair, becoming a beacon of hope.

Tony faced several obstacles along the way that tried his willpower and character strength. It was a long and difficult journey to recovery. His lack of legs was a significant physical challenge that would take years of therapy and rehabilitation to overcome.

However, the emotional wounds from his horrific past proved to be the hardest to heal, clouding his early existence with uncertainty and terror.

Tony experienced a wave of contradictory feelings as he started his healing process, including anxiety for the future, grief over the loss of his innocence, and rage at the unfairness of his circumstances.

However, among the chaos, there was a glimmer of optimism—the conviction that, whatever how bleak the night may appear, there is always hope for light at the end of the tunnel.

Tony started the difficult and protracted process of starting over with his adopted family's unconditional embrace. The physical challenge of the upcoming journey was immense; each stride was an effort to overcome pain and exhaustion, demonstrating his unwavering resolve and fortitude.

However, the most challenging aspect of his trauma to deal with was the emotional toll it took, which clouded his early existence with uncertainty and worry.

Tony took comfort in the basic pleasures of childhood throughout the early stages of his recuperation: engaging in play with toys, discovering his surroundings, and spending quality time with his loved ones.

But as he got older, the burden of his impairment started to wear him down and sowed doubt and fear in his thoughts. Would his mobility ever return? Would his classmates ever accept him? These doubts threatened to put out the optimism that blazed in his youthful heart. They were a heavy burden.

But as time went on, he developed a renewed feeling of will to overcome the obstacles and regain his freedom.

Tony started to take cautious steps towards his objective with the help of his family and the direction of his medical team, pushing himself farther every day. Even though his progress was sluggish and full with obstacles, he didn't let it stop him since he knew that each step he took would bring him one step closer to his goals.

Tony developed a stronger feeling of confidence and self-worth along with his physical power. His disability was no longer a defining factor for him; instead, he celebrated his special skills and abilities, beaming brilliantly in a world that had before looked so gloomy and unsettling.

Tony's spirit got stronger with every accomplishment and challenge faced; he is a living example of the strength of tenacity and fortitude in the face of difficulty.

However, Tony had to overcome several obstacles on his long and difficult journey to recovery. On certain days, the agony was unfathomable, and he felt as though dread and uncertainty would swallow him whole.

But at his lowest points, he found bravery in his family's love and support, and strength in their unfailing faith in his capacity to conquer the biggest challenges.

Tony found himself on the verge of a fresh start, one full of opportunity and promise, as his recuperation journey came to a conclusion. He confronted the long and unknown path ahead with the same hope and resolve that had gotten him through his worst moments. And as he walked cautiously into this strange new world for the first time, he knew that he would meet any obstacles head-on with the same bravery and tenacity that had gotten him this far.

Tony Hudgell saw his route to recovery as a symbol of the human spirit's ability to triumph over the most formidable challenges rather than just a purely physical one.

And with a sense of pride and thankfulness, he reflected on the hardships that had moulded him into the person he had become, seeing that each obstacle had served as a springboard to his great success.

# A Vision for the Future: Tony's Inspiring Mission

In the heart of West Malling, Kent, a young boy's dream takes flight, pushed by a spirit as resilient as it is vast. Tony Hudgell, with his infectious smile and unwavering drive, stands at the forefront of a movement that seeks to turn tragedy into victory, pain into purpose.

Born into a world tainted by cruelty and suffering, he has faced more difficulty in his short life than most will ever face. Yet, far from being defined by his past, Tony has emerged as a beacon of hope – a figure of strength and perseverance in the face of hardship.

As Tony thinks on the trip that has brought him to this moment, he is filled with a sense of gratitude and awe. Though the road has been long and difficult, marked by countless challenges and failures, he knows that every barrier has been a stepping stone on the path to his final goal – to make a difference in the lives of others who have suffered as he has suffered.

From a young age, Tony knew that he was meant for success. Though his goals may have seemed out of reach at times, he never wavered in his belief that he was meant for something more – something bigger than the sum of his parts.

With the steadfast support of his new family, he set out to turn his dreams into reality, one small step at a time.

For Tony, the journey towards his vision for the future started with a simple yet profound understanding – that his story had the power to inspire others to endure in the face of adversity.

Though the scars of his past may never fully heal, he knew that they could serve as a source of strength and resolve for those who were still fighting to find their way.

With this purpose firmly entrenched in his heart, Tony set out to make a change in the world around him. Through his foundation, fittingly called the Tony Hudgell

Foundation, he tried to raise awareness of the situation of mistreated and neglected children, putting a light on the darkness that so often goes unchecked in our society. Through funding events and publicity campaigns, he wanted to provide a glimmer of hope to those who had lost their way, giving them a lifeline in their darkest hour.

But Tony's vision for the future went far beyond mere charity work; he dreamed of a world in which every child could grow up feeling loved, respected, and safe.

With this goal in mind, he went on a mission to change the way society views and treats its most vulnerable members, pushing for greater understanding and responsibility in the fight against child abuse and neglect.

As Tony's power grew, so too did his effect on the world around him. From local communities to global crowds, his message of hope and resilience connected with people from all walks of life, inspiring them to stand up and make a difference in their own communities.

Through his tireless efforts and unwavering determination, he began to see the seeds of change take root, as people and groups alike rallied behind his cause.

But perhaps the most inspiring part of Tony's mission is not the effect he has had on the world, but the transformation he has undergone himself. From a young boy trying to find his place in the world, he has emerged as a confident and caring leader – a voice for the voiceless, a champion for the oppressed. With each passing day, he gets stronger and more determined, fueled by a sense of purpose that knows no limits.

As Tony looks towards the future, he does so with a sense of hope and energy, knowing that the best is yet to come. Though the road ahead may be long and fraught with challenges, he faces it with the same courage and perseverance that have taken him this far. For in his heart burns a fire that cannot be quenched – a desire for making the world a better place, one small act of kindness at a time.

In the end, Tony's idea for the future is not just about changing the world – it's about changing people. With every smile he brings to a child's face, every dollar he raises for a worthwhile cause, he moves one step closer to realizing his dream of a world where no child is left behind, where every person has the chance to grow and succeed.

And as he continues on his journey, he does so with the knowledge that he is not alone – that he is part of a global community of thinkers and doers, joined in their goal to make the world a brighter, more compassionate place for generations to come.

# Conclusion: Tony's Unstoppable Spirit

As the sun sets on another day in West Malling, Kent, the story of Tony Hudgell continues to unfold, a testament to the power of the human spirit to beat even the greatest of hurdles. Born into a world tainted by violence and suffering, Tony's journey has been marked by trials and tribulations that would have broken lesser minds. But through it all, his spirit has stayed unbroken – a beacon of hope in a world too often wrapped in darkness.

From the ashes of disaster came a young boy with a heart as brave as it is compassionate, a soul that refuses to be defined by the scars of his past. With each passing challenge, Tony has risen to the occasion, his unwavering drive and boundless positivity serving as a source of inspiration to all who know his story.

As we think on Tony's journey, we are reminded of the power of resilience and determination in the face of hardship. Though the road has been long and fraught with challenges, Tony has faced each hurdle with grit and grace, refusing to let his circumstances define his future.

From learning to walk again after the loss of his legs to fighting for the rights of abused and neglected children, he has shown us what it means to be truly invincible.

But perhaps the most inspiring part of Tony's journey is not the obstacles he has overcome, but the person he has become in the process. From a young boy trying to find his place in the world, he has emerged as a leader and a role model – a testament to the transformative power of hope and drive.

As Tony looks towards the future, he does so with a sense of hope and energy, knowing that the best is yet to come. Though the road ahead may be long and unclear, he faces it with the same guts and resilience that have brought him this far.

For in his heart burns a fire that cannot be quenched – a desire for making the world a better place, one small act of kindness at a time.

In the end, Tony's journey serves as a powerful reminder of the resilience of the human spirit – a light of hope in a world too often marred by sadness.

Though the road may be rocky and the way may be steep, Tony tells us that with courage, drive, and unwavering optimism, anything is possible.

As we say farewell to Tony and his amazing journey, let us take his spirit with us – a guiding light in the darkness, a reflection that no matter how daunting the task may seem, we are never truly alone.

And as we face our own trials and tribulations, may we take strength from his example, knowing that with the same unstoppable spirit that lives within us all, we too can overcome the odds and achieve our dreams.